# TYPE 2 DIABETES EXPLAINED EASY

Understanding Type 2 Diabetes: A Simple Guide to Causes, Symptoms, Diagnosis, Treatment, Diet, Prevention, Medications, Management & Answers to FAQs

# Rosa Andrews

# INTRODUCTION

# CHAPTER 1

# CHAPTER 2

# CHAPTER 3

# CHAPTER 4

## MEDICATIONS AND TREATMENT OPTIONS FOR TYPE 2 DIABETES

Oral Medications for Type 2 Diabetes

Insulin Therapy for Type 2 Diabetes

Other Medical Treatments for Type 2 Diabetes

Complementary and Alternative Therapies

# CHAPTER 5

## MONITORING AND MANAGING COMPLICATIONS

Monitoring Blood Sugar Levels

Managing Low and High Blood Sugar

Understanding and Preventing Diabetic Complications

# CHAPTER 6

## LIVING WITH TYPE 2 DIABETES

Building a Support System

Coping with Emotional Challenges:

Preparing for Emergencies

# CHAPTER 7

## PREVENTION AND EARLY DETECTION

Early Detection and Prevention of Complications

Making Lifestyle Changes for Better Health

# CHAPTER 8

## ANSWERS POPULAR FAQS ABOUT TYPE 2 DIABETES

I. What is Type 2 Diabetes?

II. Who is at Risk of Developing Type 2 Diabetes?

III. What Causes Type 2 Diabetes?

IV. How is Type 2 Diabetes Diagnosed?

V. What Are the Symptoms of Type 2 Diabetes?

VI. How Can Type 2 Diabetes be Treated?

VII. How Can Type 2 Diabetes be Prevented?

VIII. What Are the Complications of Type 2 Diabetes?

IX. How Do I Manage Type 2 Diabetes?

X. Can Type 2 Diabetes be cured?

# CONCLUSION

Glossary

# INTRODUCTION

Millions of individuals around the world are impacted by the chronic health issue of type 2 diabetes.

It is a condition in which your body is unable to properly use and store glucose, which is the main source of energy for your cells.

Over time, this can lead to high blood sugar levels and serious health problems.

If you have been diagnosed with type 2 diabetes, you may be feeling overwhelmed and unsure of what to do next.

However, it is important to know that with the right treatment and lifestyle changes, it is possible to effectively manage type 2 diabetes and maintain a healthy, active lifestyle.

In this book, we will take an in-depth look at type 2 diabetes, exploring its causes and risk factors, symptoms, and impact on overall health.

We will also discuss diagnosis and testing, and the various treatment options available to manage type 2 diabetes, including lifestyle changes, medications, and complementary and alternative therapies.

Throughout this guide, you will find practical tips and advice for monitoring and managing your blood sugar levels, preventing complications, and living well with type 2 diabetes.

Despite being a common condition, many people are still unsure about what type 2 diabetes is, what causes it, and what the risk factors are.

. In this chapter, we will provide an overview of type 2 diabetes, including its causes and risk factors, to help you better understand this condition and what you can do to manage it.

# What is Type 2 Diabetes?

Type 2 diabetes is a metabolic condition that arises when the body either becomes resistant to insulin or the pancreas is unable to produce enough insulin to maintain proper blood sugar level.

Insulin is a hormone that helps to transport glucose from the blood into the cells, where it is used for energy.

When insulin resistance or a lack of insulin production occurs, glucose builds up in the blood, leading to high blood sugar levels.

Over time, high blood sugar levels can cause damage to the body, including nerve damage, vision problems, kidney disease, and an increased risk of heart disease and stroke.

# Causes of Type 2 Diabetes

The exact cause of type 2 diabetes is not fully understood, but several factors can contribute to its development. These include:

Insulin resistance: As mentioned, insulin resistance occurs when the cells in the body become less responsive to insulin, making it difficult for the hormone to regulate blood sugar levels.

This can result in elevated blood sugar levels and a heightened risk of type 2 diabetes.

**Pancreatic beta cell dysfunction:** The beta cells in the pancreas are responsible for producing insulin.

If the beta cells are not functioning properly, they may not produce enough insulin to regulate blood sugar levels, leading to type 2 diabetes.

**Genetics:** Family history and genetics can also play a role in the development of type 2 diabetes.

If you have a family history of type 2 diabetes, your chances of developing the condition may be higher.

**Obesity:** Obesity, especially abdominal obesity, can contribute to the development of type 2 diabetes.

This is because excess weight can lead to insulin resistance and a reduction in insulin production.

**Lack of physical activity:** Physical inactivity can also increase the risk of type 2 diabetes, as it can lead to insulin resistance and decreased insulin production.

# Risk Factors for Type 2 Diabetes

In addition to the causes of type 2 diabetes, several risk factors can increase your likelihood of developing the condition. These include:

**Age:** As people age, particularly after the age of 45, the risk of developing type 2 diabetes increases.

**Family history:** Individuals with a family history of type 2 diabetes are at a heightened risk of developing the condition.

**Ethnicity:** Certain ethnic groups, such as African Americans, Native Americans, and Hispanics, have a higher risk of developing type 2 diabetes.

**High blood pressure:** High blood pressure can increase the risk of type 2 diabetes, as it can damage the blood vessels and increase the risk of heart disease and stroke.

**Unhealthy diet:** A diet that is high in processed foods, sugar, and unhealthy fats can increase the risk of type 2 diabetes, as it can lead to weight gain and insulin resistance.

**Physical inactivity:** A sedentary lifestyle can also increase the risk of type 2 diabetes, as it can lead to weight gain and insulin resistance.

# Symptoms of Type 2 Diabetes

1.      Increased thirst and frequent urination: High blood sugar levels can lead to increased thirst and the need to urinate more frequently.

This is due to the body trying to get rid of the excess glucose by increasing fluid intake and producing more urine.

2.      Extreme hunger: When the body is unable to use glucose effectively, it will start to break down stored fat and muscle, leading to an increase in hunger.

3.      Fatigue: Excess glucose in the blood can prevent the body from effectively utilizing energy, leading to feelings of tiredness and fatigue.

4.      Blurred vision: High blood sugar levels can cause fluid to be pulled from the lenses of the eyes, leading to blurred vision.

5.      Slow wound healing: High blood sugar levels can impair circulation and reduce the body's ability to heal wounds.

6.      Tingling or numbness in the extremities: High blood sugar levels can damage the nerves, leading to tingling or numbness in the hands and feet.

7.      Skin infections: High blood sugar levels can make the skin more susceptible to infections, such as yeast infections.

8.      Unexpected weight loss: Despite increased hunger, individuals with Type 2 Diabetes may experience unexpected weight loss as the body breaks down stored fat and muscle.

9.      Dark patches on the skin: Dark, velvety patches on the skin, particularly in the armpits and neck, can be a sign of insulin resistance, a risk factor for Type 2 Diabetes.

10.      Frequent infections: High blood sugar levels can weaken the immune system, making individuals more susceptible to infections.

It is important to note that not all individuals with Type 2 Diabetes will experience all of these symptoms.

Some individuals may experience only a few of these symptoms, while others may not experience any symptoms at all.

Regular check-ups with a healthcare provider can help detect the condition early and prevent the onset of complications.

In conclusion, Type 2 Diabetes is a serious health condition that affects millions of people around the world. It is important to be aware of the causes and risk factors for developing the condition, such as a family history of diabetes, being overweight, and leading a sedentary lifestyle.

By taking steps to reduce these risk factors and managing their diet, exercise, and stress levels, individuals can reduce their chances of developing Type 2 Diabetes.

It is also essential for those with the condition to work closely with their healthcare provider to create a treatment plan that is tailored to their individual needs. This may include lifestyle changes, medications, and regular monitoring of blood glucose levels.

In short, Type 2 Diabetes is a manageable condition that requires a combination of lifestyle changes and medical management.

With the right support and care, individuals with Type 2 Diabetes can lead full and active lives while keeping their condition under control.

# CHAPTER 1

## Understanding Type 2 Diabetes

### *How Type 2 Diabetes Affects the Body*

Type 2 diabetes is a chronic condition that affects how the body processes glucose, or sugar, the main source of energy for our cells.

When someone has type 2 diabetes, their body either resists the effects of insulin or doesn't produce enough of it. As a result, glucose accumulates in the bloodstream instead of being taken into the cells, leading to high blood sugar levels.

Over time, high blood sugar levels can cause damage to many parts of the body, including the heart, blood vessels, eyes, kidneys, and nerves.

*Here are some of the most common ways that type 2 diabetes affects the body:*

1. Heart and Blood Vessels: High blood sugar levels can cause a buildup of fat in the blood vessels, leading to an increased risk of heart disease and stroke.

2. Eyes: High blood sugar levels can cause damage to the blood vessels in the eyes, leading to a condition called diabetic retinopathy. If left untreated, diabetic retinopathy can cause vision loss or blindness.

3. Kidneys: High blood sugar levels can cause damage to the blood vessels in the kidneys, leading to a condition called diabetic nephropathy.

If left untreated, diabetic nephropathy can lead to kidney failure.

4. Nerves: High blood sugar levels can cause damage to the nerves, leading to a condition called diabetic neuropathy.

Diabetic neuropathy can cause numbness, tingling, or burning sensations in the hands and feet.

## Comparing Type 1 and Type 2 Diabetes

Type 1 and type 2 diabetes are two different types of diabetes, but they share some similarities.

Both types of diabetes cause high blood sugar levels and can lead to serious health complications.

However, there are some key differences between type 1 and type 2 diabetes.

# 1. Causes:

Type 1 diabetes is caused by an autoimmune response that destroys the insulin-producing cells in the pancreas.

On the other hand, type 2 diabetes is caused by a combination of factors, including a family history of diabetes, being overweight, and leading a sedentary lifestyle.

# 2. Age of Onset:

Type 1 diabetes usually develops in childhood or adolescence, while type 2 diabetes usually develops in adulthood.

# 3. Treatment:

Type 1 diabetes requires daily injections of insulin or the use of an insulin pump.

On the other hand, type 2 diabetes can be managed through lifestyle changes, such as diet and exercise, and oral medications or insulin injections if necessary.

# The Impact of Type 2 Diabetes on Overall Health

Type 2 diabetes can have a significant impact on a person's overall health, leading to serious health complications and a decreased quality of life.

*Here are some of the most common impacts of type 2 diabetes on overall health:*

**1. Decreased Quality of Life:** Type 2 diabetes can cause a wide range of physical and emotional symptoms, including fatigue, mood swings, and sexual dysfunction.

**2. Increased Risk of Health Complications:** Type 2 diabetes can increase the risk of serious health complications, such as heart disease, stroke, kidney disease, and blindness.

**3. Increased Healthcare Costs:** Type 2 diabetes can also increase healthcare costs, as it often requires ongoing medical care and treatment for complications.

People with type 2 diabetes need to manage their condition and make lifestyle changes to prevent or delay the onset of health complications.

This includes eating a healthy diet, staying physically active, and taking medication as prescribed.

By working with their healthcare team, people with type 2 diabetes can maintain their health and prevent serious health complications.

# CHAPTER 2

## Diagnosis and Testing For Type 2 Diabetes

Diagnosing and testing for type 2 diabetes is a critical aspect of managing the disease effectively.

It is important to understand the various screening and diagnostic tests that are available for individuals who are suspected of having type 2 diabetes.

In this chapter, we will discuss the different methods for screening for type 2 diabetes and the various diagnostic tests that are used to confirm the diagnosis.

# Screening for Type 2 Diabetes

Type 2 diabetes is a common condition, affecting millions of people around the world.

It is often asymptomatic in its early stages, which makes it difficult to detect without proper screening. Screening for type 2 diabetes is typically done through a simple blood test that measures your fasting blood glucose levels. T

his test is usually done in the morning before you have had anything to eat or drink. If your fasting blood glucose levels are higher than normal, it may indicate the presence of type 2 diabetes.

## Diagnostic Tests for Type 2 Diabetes

*Several diagnostic tests are used to confirm the diagnosis of type 2 diabetes. These tests include:*

# Oral Glucose Tolerance Test (OGTT)

The OGTT is a test that measures your blood glucose levels after you have consumed a sugary drink.

This test is typically done two hours after drinking the sugary drink, and it helps to determine if you have type 2 diabetes by measuring your body's ability to handle glucose.

# A1C Test

The A1C test measures your average blood glucose levels over the past two to three months.

This test is a simple blood test that can be done in your doctor's office or at home. A1C test results are expressed as a percentage, and a result of 6.5% or higher is considered to be indicative of type 2 diabetes.

# Fructosamine Test

The fructosamine test is a test that measures your average blood glucose levels over the past one to three weeks. This test is typically done in conjunction with other diagnostic tests, and it provides a more detailed picture of your blood glucose control.

# _Understanding A1C and Other Test Results_

The A1C test and other diagnostic tests for type 2 diabetes are important tools that help you and your doctor to understand your blood glucose control and how well your treatment plan is working.

It is important to understand the results of these tests and what they mean for your health.

For example, an A1C result of 6.5% or higher is considered to be indicative of type 2 diabetes, while a result of 7% or higher may indicate poor blood glucose control.

Other test results, such as fructosamine levels, can provide a more detailed picture of your blood glucose control over a specific period.

In conclusion, screening and diagnostic tests for type 2 diabetes are critical tools for managing the disease effectively.

It is important to understand these tests, what they measure, and what the results mean for your health.

By working closely with your doctor and regularly monitoring your blood glucose levels, you can help to ensure that you are effectively managing your type 2 diabetes and maintaining good overall health.

# CHAPTER 3

## Lifestyle Changes for Managing Type 2 Diabetes

As someone living with Type 2 Diabetes, making lifestyle changes can be a significant challenge. However, these changes are necessary to help manage the condition and prevent the onset of serious health problems.

We'll discuss the various lifestyle changes that can help you effectively manage Type 2 Diabetes.

# Healthy Eating and Meal Planning:

One of the most important lifestyle changes you can make to manage Type 2 Diabetes is to adopt a healthy eating plan.

This includes consuming more whole grains, fruits, and vegetables and reducing your intake of added sugars and unhealthy fats.

It's also essential to manage your portion sizes and eat regular, well-balanced meals throughout the day.

For example, a person with Type 2 Diabetes can start their day with a bowl of oatmeal, add a serving of fruit, and have a salad with grilled chicken for lunch. In the evening, they can have a vegetable stir-fry with brown rice.

## Type 2 Diabetes Food List

It is important for individuals with type 2 diabetes to be mindful of their food choices and maintain a balanced, nutritious diet.

Let's explore the type 2 diabetes food list, including what foods to eat and what to avoid to help manage blood sugar levels and maintain overall health.

One of the key components of a healthy diet for individuals with type 2 diabetes is to focus on nutrient-dense, low-glycemic foods.

These include whole grains, fiber-rich fruits and vegetables, lean protein, and healthy fats such as nuts, seeds, and avocado.

These foods are not only nutritious but also help to regulate blood sugar levels and promote feelings of fullness, reducing the temptation to snack on less healthy options.

In terms of carbohydrates, it is recommended to choose whole grains such as brown rice, quinoa, and whole-wheat bread instead of refined carbohydrates such as white bread and pasta.

These whole grains are a good source of fiber, which helps slow down the digestion and absorption of carbohydrates, keeping blood sugar levels stable.

It is also recommended to include a variety of colorful fruits and vegetables in the diet, as they are rich in vitamins, minerals, and fiber, and have a low glycemic index.

When it comes to protein, it is important to choose lean sources such as chicken, fish, and beans.

These foods not only provide important nutrients but also help to regulate blood sugar levels and promote feelings of fullness.

On the other hand, it is best to limit processed meats, such as sausages and bacon, as they can be high in saturated fat and salt, which can contribute to a number of health problems.

Healthy fats are also an important part of a type 2 diabetes food list.

Foods such as nuts, seeds, avocados, and olive oil contain unsaturated fats that have been shown to have numerous health benefits.

These healthy fats can help regulate blood sugar levels, reduce inflammation, and improve heart health.

On the other hand, it is important to limit unhealthy fats such as those found in fried foods and processed snacks, as they can contribute to high cholesterol and other health problems.

In addition to focusing on nutrient-dense, low-glycemic foods, it is also important to limit portion sizes and be mindful of food and drink choices.

This may include reducing sugar-sweetened beverages, limiting processed snacks, and avoiding high-calorie foods that are high in sugar and unhealthy fats.

# Physical Activity and Exercise

Exercise is another crucial component of managing Type 2 Diabetes.

Regular physical activity helps to lower blood sugar levels, improve insulin sensitivity, and reduce the risk of heart disease and other related health problems.

For instance, a person with Type 2 Diabetes can aim for at least 30 minutes of moderate-intensity physical activity, such as brisk walking, every day.

If you are just starting out, start with 10-15 minute increments and gradually build up over time.

# Managing Stress & Sleep

Stress and sleep are also essential factors in managing Type 2 Diabetes.

Stress can cause hormonal changes that increase blood sugar levels, while lack of sleep can lead to decreased insulin sensitivity.

To reduce stress, try practicing relaxation techniques, such as deep breathing and meditation.

Aim for 7-9 hours of sleep per night, and establish a consistent bedtime routine to help you fall asleep faster.

In conclusion, managing Type 2 Diabetes requires a combination of lifestyle changes, including healthy eating and meal planning, physical activity and exercise, stress management, and adequate sleep.

By making these changes, you can improve your overall health and effectively manage your condition.

Remember to work closely with your healthcare provider to develop a personalized plan that works best for you. With time, patience, and commitment, you can successfully manage Type 2 Diabetes and live a healthy and fulfilling life.

# CHAPTER 4

## Medications and Treatment Options for Type 2 Diabetes

Type 2 diabetes is a chronic condition that affects the way your body processes glucose, a type of sugar that provides energy for your cells.

If left unmanaged, it can lead to serious health problems, including heart disease, stroke, and nerve damage.

The good news is that with proper care and management, it is possible to effectively control your blood sugar levels and reduce your risk of complications.

One of the key components of managing type 2 diabetes is medication.

There are several different types of medications and treatments available, each with its own unique set of benefits and risks.

These are some of the most common medications and treatment options available for type 2 diabetes:

## *Oral Medications for Type 2 Diabetes*

Oral medications for type 2 diabetes work by helping your body use insulin more effectively or by reducing the amount of glucose produced by your liver.

Examples of these medications include metformin, sulfonylureas, and DPP-4 inhibitors.

These medications can help improve your blood sugar control and prevent complications, but they may also cause side effects, such as low blood sugar or weight gain.

# Insulin Therapy for Type 2 Diabetes

If your body is no longer able to produce enough insulin on its own, or if oral medications are no longer effective, your doctor may recommend insulin therapy.

Insulin is a hormone that helps your body use glucose for energy.

There are several different types of insulin available, including rapid-acting, long-acting, and combination formulations.

Your doctor will work with you to determine the best type of insulin and dosing schedule for your needs.

# _Other Medical Treatments for Type 2 Diabetes_

In addition to oral medications and insulin therapy, there are other medical treatments available for type 2 diabetes, including GLP-1 receptor agonists, SGLT2 inhibitors, and sodium-glucose cotransporter 2 (SGLT2) inhibitors. These medications work in different ways to help improve your blood sugar control, but they may also cause side effects, such as gastrointestinal distress or urinary tract infections.

# _Complementary and Alternative Therapies_

While there is limited evidence to support the use of complementary and alternative therapies for type 2 diabetes, some people may find them helpful in managing their condition.

Examples of these therapies include acupuncture, herbal supplements, and mindfulness-based stress reduction. However, it's important to talk to your doctor before trying any complementary or alternative therapies, as they may interact with your medications or other medical treatments.

In conclusion, there are several different medications and treatment options available for type 2 diabetes, each with its own set of benefits and risks.

Your doctor will work with you to determine the best course of treatment based on your individual needs and health status.

Whether you're taking oral medications, insulin, or exploring complementary and alternative therapies, the most important thing is to stick to your treatment plan and make lifestyle changes that support your overall health and well-being.

# CHAPTER 5

## Monitoring and Managing Complications

Monitoring and managing diabetes is essential to prevent these complications and ensure that you stay healthy.

Let's discuss the importance of monitoring blood sugar levels, managing low and high blood sugar, and understanding and preventing diabetic complications.

## *Monitoring Blood Sugar Levels*

Monitoring blood sugar levels is a crucial aspect of managing type 2 diabetes.

Keeping a close eye on your blood sugar levels helps you make informed decisions about how to adjust your diet, exercise, and medication regimen.

A simple and convenient way to monitor your blood sugar levels is by using a glucometer.

This device measures the amount of glucose in your blood and gives you an instant reading.

You can use it to check your blood sugar levels at various times of the day, such as before and after meals, to see how your diet, exercise, and medication regimen is impacting your blood sugar levels.

# Managing Low and High Blood Sugar

Low blood sugar levels, also known as hypoglycemia, can be a dangerous and even life-threatening complication of type 2 diabetes. Low blood sugar levels occur when your blood sugar drops too low, causing you to experience symptoms such as dizziness, confusion, sweating, and even loss of consciousness.

To prevent low blood sugar levels, it is important to eat regularly, monitor your blood sugar levels, and adjust your medication and physical activity accordingly.

If you experience symptoms of low blood sugar levels, it is important to eat or drink something that contains sugar, such as fruit juice or candy, to quickly raise your blood sugar levels.

High blood sugar levels, also known as hyperglycemia, can also be a serious complication of type 2 diabetes.

High blood sugar levels can damage your body over time and increase your risk of developing long-term complications, such as heart disease, eye problems, and nerve damage.

To prevent high blood sugar levels, it is important to maintain a healthy diet, exercise regularly, and take your medication as prescribed.

If your blood sugar levels are consistently high, it may be necessary to adjust your medication or lifestyle habits to better manage your condition.

# Understanding and Preventing Diabetic Complications

Type 2 diabetes can increase your risk of developing a range of long-term complications, including heart disease, eye problems, nerve damage, and kidney disease. To prevent these complications, it is important to manage your blood sugar levels effectively and adopt a healthy lifestyle.

This includes maintaining a healthy diet, exercising regularly, getting enough sleep, managing stress, and taking your medication as prescribed.

Regular check-ups with your healthcare provider can also help you detect and treat any potential complications early on, so you can take action to prevent further damage to your body.

In conclusion, monitoring and managing blood sugar levels, preventing low and high blood sugar, and understanding and preventing diabetic complications are all essential aspects of managing type 2 diabetes.

By working closely with your healthcare provider, following a healthy lifestyle, and staying informed about your condition, you can effectively manage your type 2 diabetes and reduce your risk of developing long-term complications.

# CHAPTER 6

## LIVING WITH TYPE 2 DIABETES

We all know how serious and long-term a diagnosis of type 2 diabetes can be.

It's a condition that will require a lifetime of diligent care and attention. With the right treatments, lifestyle modifications, and support system, however, it is possible to live a normal and healthy life with type 2 diabetes

While it can be managed with proper care, it is not an easy road to navigate.

However, with the right tools and support, those with type 2 diabetes can lead full and healthy lives.

We will explore various ways to live with type 2 diabetes, including building a support system, coping with emotional challenges, staying motivated and adhering to treatment, and preparing for emergencies.

# Building a Support System

Living with type 2 diabetes can be overwhelming and isolating, but having a strong support system can make all the difference.

Whether it's family, friends, or a support group, having someone to turn to for advice, encouragement, and comfort can be invaluable.

A support system can also help you stay on track with your treatment plan and keep you motivated to make healthy choices.

Having a support system and a team of people who understand and can provide guidance, advice, and encouragement is an invaluable part of managing diabetes.

Whether it's a family member, a close friend, or a medical professional, having a support system can provide you with the resources to handle the challenges that come with living with type 2 diabetes.

It might be difficult to put yourself out there and ask for help, as many people feel like they have to go through it alone, however, it can be an incredibly rewarding experience once you've found a supportive and understanding network of individuals.

The first step towards establishing a support system for type 2 diabetes is to connect with others.

You should look to find all types of people in your network who can provide support, whether it's for your physical health, mental health, dietary and exercise changes, or to help you find ways to take medications. For family support, look to parents and siblings, as well as aunts, uncles, and cousins that might have similar experiences and can share useful advice.

It's also important to find friends and colleagues who are understanding and willing to listen, who you can turn to if times get difficult.

And, of course, there are numerous diabetes support groups around the country- and more on the internet- that can provide valuable insight and information on how to best manage the condition.

Joining one of these groups can be a great way to meet others who are facing the same difficulties and who can provide emotional support.

Additionally, the medical professionals who are part of your care team should help to form the basis of your support system throughout your journey with type 2 diabetes.

This could include your primary care doctor and any specialists on your team. Knowing these people have your back may give you peace of mind that you are on the right track in managing your diabetes.

Research studies have shown that having regular contact with a diabetes team can cause a reduction in hospitalizations and A1C readings.

It's also important to make sure that these medical professionals have the most up-to-date information about you so that they can provide the best possible care.

In the end, establishing a strong support system for managing type 2 diabetes is essential for succeeding in the journey.

It can provide emotional relief in difficult times and help to keep you on track with managing your diabetes in the long run. So, if you're living with type 2 diabetes, don't be afraid to ask for help- as it can be the difference between feeling alone in this journey and feeling like you have a team of individuals to lean on in your corner.

# Coping with Emotional Challenges:

Managing type 2 diabetes can bring up a range of emotions, including frustration, fear, and anxiety. It's important to understand and acknowledge these feelings and find healthy ways to cope with them. Talking to a trusted friend or family member, seeing a therapist, or participating in a support group can all help you manage your emotions.

It's also important to find healthy ways to manage stress, such as exercise, meditation, or hobbies.

As such, it can be easy to become overwhelmed with guilt and feel powerless in the face of the condition.

It can also be hard to hold oneself accountable for the changes necessary to manage the condition, and consequently lead to feelings of frustration, guilt, and depression.

It is important to remember that Diabetes is a real medical condition, and as such, must be managed in the same way one would manage any medical condition.

Dealing with the emotional aspects of living with diabetes can seem to be a heavy burden, but there are several ways in which emotional well-being can be developed and maintained.

Unsurprisingly, emotional well-being is linked to physical health, especially when it comes to type 2 diabetes.

The emotional capacity to manage diabetes is just as important as being able to follow doctors' orders when it comes to managing the condition.

It is important to stay as positive as possible. Taking a moment to express your concerns, speaking to friends who understand the condition, and listening to expert advice can all help to de-stress and boost morale.

Developing realistic goals and understanding one's limits can also alleviate feelings of guilt and pressure.

Regular exercise is also beneficial not just for physical health, but also for mental health; physical activity has been proven to be a great way to help manage stress and those who are more physically active tend to report having higher self-esteem and improved quality of life.

It is also important to take an active interest in your healthcare. Making sure you schedule routine doctor's appointments and checking blood sugar levels regularly, as well as learning about proper nutrition and therapies, can all help to reduce feelings of frustration.

Keeping records of your progress can also be beneficial and provide purpose and structure to managing the condition.

Having the support of professionals and family can also be a huge benefit psychologically, as well as providing practical care like assisting with medicine and diet management.

Support groups are also a great way to restore feelings of self-efficacy and find comfort in the company of others. Being around people who understand the condition and can relate to one's struggles can be invaluable in aiding emotional health.

Reaching out to individuals online or in person who has struggled with type 2 diabetes can also be a great source of understanding and empathy.

Additionally, professional counseling can also be a helpful resource to aid in dealing with the emotional aspects of type 2 diabetes.

Living with type 2 diabetes can be an emotional challenge, but it is important to remember that there are many ways to effectively cope with the condition. Taking an active role in one's healthcare, staying positive, reaching out to sources of support, and speaking to professionals can all help manage the emotional burden of managing the condition.

Staying Motivated and Adhering to Treatment

Staying motivated and sticking to your treatment plan is key to managing type 2 diabetes. It can be tempting to skip medication or make unhealthy choices, but it's important to remember the long-term consequences of not adhering to your treatment. Find what works for you, whether it's setting small, achievable goals, finding a workout buddy, or rewarding yourself for sticking to your plan.

Living with type 2 diabetes can present many challenges, so it is crucial to stay motivated and adhere to treatment. This can be easier said than done when facing the physical, mental, and emotional difficulties this chronic condition can bring, so taking the necessary steps to remain motivated and stick to your treatment plan is key in managing the condition.

One of the most important factors for staying motivated is having a positive and helpful attitude about type 2 diabetes and how it impacts your life.

Accepting the situation and understanding how to manage it will make it easier to stay motivated and committed to a healthier lifestyle.

Knowing that you are in control and grateful that you can make changes to improve your well-being is paramount in staying inspired.

Another tool for staying motivated is to focus on the positive. Throughout treatment and management, there may be times when your condition seems to be regressing.

During these times, it can be easy to dwell on the sense of failure and discouragement.

A good way to keep yourself motivated is to focus on what you can achieve and be proud of with daily constructive changes.

Celebrate your victories and celebrate every step, no matter how small, towards a healthier lifestyle.

For example, if you can stick to a dietary change for a whole week, reward yourself with a movie, a night out, or a delicious treat.

Setting realistic goals and a clear plan of action is another great way of staying motivated.

It is essential to remember that change takes time, so have realistic expectations and understand that it can take time to adjust to a new lifestyle.

Breaking your journey into manageable steps with achievable goals will help you stay on track, so make sure to set achievable goals and celebrate the milestones you reach.

It is also important to remember that staying motivated and adhering to treatment can come easier with some additional support.

Seek out a community where you can get the motivation, support, and understanding of people in the same situation.

Reach out to family and friends and discuss your goals with them.

Having a support system of those closest to you will give you the assurance and reassurance you need during times of difficulty.

Sticking with a regular exercise routine is another great way of keeping you focused, motivated, and in shape. Daily physical activity not only helps regulate your blood sugar levels, but it can also be a great source of emotional relief and an effective means for stress relief. Plus it can help keep your focus on the positives and boosts your morale.

A routine of physical activity can also help to reduce your risk of developing serious complications from type 2 diabetes.

Staying motivated and adhering to treatment is key in managing type 2 diabetes, but it can also be a difficult task to maintain.

The key is to focus on the positives, set achievable goals and create a plan of action, have a supportive network of family and friends, and remember to have some fun and move around.

Taking these steps will help you become the best version of yourself and live your life with type 2 diabetes.

# Preparing for Emergencies

When you are living with Type 2 diabetes, it is important to plan for emergencies.

Emergencies can happen and it is important to be prepared.

Emergencies can range from minor inconveniences to life-threatening events.

A few key tips for preparing for emergencies may include having an updated list of all medications, carrying an emergency supply of food, establishing a support network and asking for help when it is needed, knowing where the nearest medical facility is, and creating a diabetes emergency kit.

It is important to maintain an updated list of medications. Keeping a list of all appropriate medications, including insulin, glucose monitors, and medical supplies, can help ensure that the medications are readily available during an emergency.

Having a record of all medications, dosages, and dispositions of medications can be important to provide to first responders or health care practitioners, who may not be familiar with the patient's treatment approach.

Having an emergency supply of food is also important. People with diabetes will generally require snacks throughout the day, to maintain and control their blood glucose.

If a person is traveling, they should have a source of snacks, such as protein bars, nuts, or other items that do not require refrigeration. In the event of an emergency, having a non-perishable food supply can help maintain blood glucose and prevent hypoglycemia.

Having a support network is also important for type 2 diabetes.

Being able to reach out and ask for help as needed can be the difference between life and death. Developing relationships with family, friends, and neighbors in the community can be beneficial.

Not only can a support network help in times of emergency but having a network of people to rely on for emotional and physical support can be invaluable.

Planning for emergencies should also include knowing where the nearest medical facility is located.

Knowing the locations of local hospitals, treatment centers, and pharmacies can be critical in an emergency. For individuals who live alone, having contacts to help in an emergency can be especially important.

Finally, having a diabetic medical emergency kit can be helpful.

A medical emergency kit should include a list of medications, syringes, cotton swabs, and a glucometer. Additionally, packets of sugar-free juice, glucose tablets, and candy bars should be kept in an accessible location. Items in a medical emergency kit are typically replaced every year, as medications and dosages may change over time.

Living with type 2 diabetes often requires extra planning and preparation.

Preparing for emergencies can help reduce the risk of major health complications occurring.

Keeping an updated list of medications, establishing a support network, knowing the location of the nearest medical facilities, and creating a diabetic medical emergency kit are key steps for preparing for emergencies. By planning, individuals with type 2 diabetes can rest assured that they are prepared.

Conclusion: Living with type 2 diabetes can be challenging, but with the right support and tools, it is possible to manage and thrive.

Building a support system, coping with emotional challenges, staying motivated, adhering to treatment, and preparing for emergencies are all important aspects of managing this condition.

By taking control of your health and seeking help when needed, you can live a fulfilling life with type 2 diabetes.

# CHAPTER 7

## Prevention and Early Detection

While it is a serious condition that requires ongoing management, the good news is that with proper care and attention, many people with type 2 diabetes can lead full and healthy lives.

This chapter will focus on the prevention and early detection of type 2 diabetes and how you can take steps to improve your health and lower your risk of developing this condition.

Preventing Type 2 Diabetes: One of the most important steps you can take to prevent type 2 diabetes is to make healthy lifestyle choices.

Eating a healthy diet, engaging in regular physical activity, and maintaining a healthy weight are all key factors in reducing your risk of developing type 2 diabetes. Additionally, quitting smoking and limiting alcohol intake can also help to lower your risk.

## _Early Detection and Prevention of Complications_

The earlier type 2 diabetes is detected, the more manageable it is, and the better chance you have of avoiding serious health problems. Regular check-ups and screenings are key to the early detection and prevention of complications.

You should also be mindful of the warning signs of type 2 diabetes, such as frequent urination, increased thirst, and blurred vision. If you experience any symptoms, it is important to see a doctor promptly.

# _Making Lifestyle Changes for Better Health_

Lifestyle changes are an important part of preventing and managing type 2 diabetes. It's important to find ways to make healthy eating, physical activity, and stress management a regular part of your life.

You can start by incorporating small changes into your daily routine, such as choosing healthier foods, walking or biking instead of driving, and taking a few minutes each day to practice mindfulness or meditation.

Making healthy lifestyle choices, such as eating a balanced diet, getting regular physical activity, and managing stress can help to lower your risk of developing type 2 diabetes.

Remember that it's never too late to make positive changes to your health, and with the right support, you can live a full and healthy life with type 2 diabetes.

# CHAPTER 8

## Answers Popular FAQs about Type 2 Diabetes

### I. What is Type 2 Diabetes?

Type 2 diabetes is a chronic condition that occurs when the pancreas either does not produce enough insulin or the body does not use insulin effectively.

It typically develops in adulthood but can also occur in children. Insulin is a hormone produced by the pancreas that helps keep blood sugar levels in check.

When insulin production is insufficient or does not work effectively, glucose cannot be absorbed into cells, so it builds up in the blood.

This increases blood sugar levels, which can lead to serious complications if left untreated.

## II. Who is at Risk of Developing Type 2 Diabetes?

People are at greater risk of developing type 2 diabetes if they are older than 45 years of age, overweight or obese, have a family history of the condition, have high blood pressure, have a sedentary lifestyle, or have a history of gestational diabetes.

## III. What Causes Type 2 Diabetes?

The exact cause of type 2 diabetes is still unknown, but it is believed to be a combination of genetic and environmental factors.

These include obesity, lack of exercise, unhealthy diet, and certain medications or illnesses.

## IV. How is Type 2 Diabetes Diagnosed?

Type 2 diabetes is typically diagnosed through a blood test known as the A1C test.

This measures the average amount of glucose in your bloodstream over the past two to three months. If the result is higher than normal, it could indicate diabetes. Your doctor may also order more specific tests such as a fasting plasma glucose test (FPG), which measures your blood sugar levels after you haven't eaten for at least 8 hours, or a two-hour oral glucose tolerance test (OGTT), which measures your blood sugar levels after you've had a sugary drink.

## V. What Are the Symptoms of Type 2 Diabetes?

The common symptoms of type 2 diabetes include increased thirst, fatigue, and frequent urination.

Other symptoms may include blurred vision, slow healing of wounds, nauseous feelings after eating, and tingling or numbness in the extremities.

## VI. How Can Type 2 Diabetes be Treated?

Type 2 diabetes can be effectively treated and managed with a combination of lifestyle changes and medication. A healthy diet, regular physical activity, avoiding smoking, and monitoring blood sugar levels are essential to effective treatment.

Your doctor may also prescribe medications such as insulin, sulfonylureas, thiazolidinediones, meglitinides, and GLP-1 agonists, depending on your individual needs.

## VII. How Can Type 2 Diabetes be Prevented?

Type 2 diabetes is often preventable by maintaining a healthy lifestyle. Eating a balanced diet, exercising regularly, and avoiding smoking are some of the key ways to prevent type 2 diabetes.

## VIII. What Are the Complications of Type 2 Diabetes?

People with type 2 diabetes are at a higher risk for developing a variety of serious conditions.

These can include stroke, high blood pressure, heart disease, nerve damage, kidney disease, and eye damage.

## IX. How Do I Manage Type 2 Diabetes?

Managing type 2 diabetes requires a combination of lifestyle changes, medication, and regular glucose monitoring. Eating a healthy diet, exercising regularly, avoiding smoking, and maintaining a healthy weight are all essential aspects of managing type 2 diabetes.

Your doctor may also prescribe medication such as insulin, sulfonylureas, thiazolidinediones, meglitinides, and GLP-1 agonists.

## X. Can Type 2 Diabetes be cured?

At the current time, there is no cure for type 2 diabetes. However, it can be managed and controlled through lifestyle changes and medication.

Controlling your blood sugar levels will help you reduce the risk of developing complications associated with type 2 diabetes.

# CONCLUSION

Living with Type 2 diabetes can be a challenging experience, but with proper management and support, individuals with the condition can lead healthy, fulfilling lives. In this book,

we have explored the various aspects of Type 2 diabetes, from understanding the condition and its causes, to managing its symptoms and complications, and making lifestyle changes to improve health.

The importance of comprehensive diabetes management cannot be overstated. Regular monitoring of blood sugar levels, taking medications as prescribed, making healthy eating and physical activity choices, and seeking treatment for emotional challenges are all crucial steps in effectively managing Type 2 diabetes.

Building a strong support system and having access to resources for ongoing support and education are also essential.

We encourage individuals living with Type 2 diabetes to be proactive in managing their condition and to seek support when needed.

With the right tools, resources, and mindset, living with Type 2 diabetes can be a positive and empowering experience.

Whether through support groups, online communities, or one-on-one support with healthcare professionals, there are many resources available for individuals to receive ongoing education and support.

In conclusion, we hope that this book has provided valuable information and insights into the management of Type 2 diabetes.

We encourage individuals to use this information to empower themselves to take control of their health, and to continue to seek out resources and support as they navigate this journey.

# Glossary

A1C: A blood test that measures average blood sugar levels over the past 2-3 months.

Blood sugar levels: The amount of glucose (sugar) in the blood.

Complications: Long-term problems that can arise from uncontrolled diabetes, such as heart disease, nerve damage, and vision problems.

Diabetes: A chronic condition in which the body is unable to produce or properly use insulin, resulting in high blood sugar levels.

Diagnostic tests: Tests used to diagnose diabetes, such as the A1C test, fasting blood glucose test, and oral glucose tolerance test.

Glucose: A type of sugar that is the main source of energy for the body.

Insulin is a hormone produced by the pancreas that helps keep blood sugar levels in check.

Lifestyle changes: Changes in diet, exercise, and other habits can help manage diabetes and improve overall health.

Medications: Drugs used to treat diabetes, including oral medications and insulin therapy.

Type 1 diabetes: A type of diabetes in which the body is unable to produce insulin.

Type 2 diabetes: A type of diabetes in which the body is unable to properly use insulin.

Walking: A low-impact form of exercise that can help improve blood sugar levels and overall health.

Printed in Great Britain
by Amazon